the
movement
therapy
deck

ALSO BY
ERICA HORNTHAL

Body Aware: Rediscover Your Mind-Body Connection, Stop Feeling Stuck, and Improve Your Mental Health with Simple Movement Practices

the movement therapy deck

52 Mindful Movement Exercises to Regulate Your Nervous System and Process Trauma

Erica Hornthal, LCPC, BC-DMT

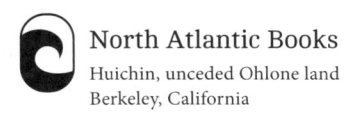

North Atlantic Books
Huichin, unceded Ohlone land
Berkeley, California

Copyright © 2024 by Erica Hornthal. All rights reserved. No portion of this book, except for brief review, may be reproduced, stored in a retrieval system, or transmitted in any form or by any means—electronic, mechanical, photocopying, recording, or otherwise—without the written permission of the publisher. For information contact North Atlantic Books.

Published by
North Atlantic Books
Huichin, unceded Ohlone land
Berkeley, California

Cover design and card art by
Jasmine Hromjak
Book design by
Happenstance Type-O-Rama

Printed in China

The Movement Therapy Deck: 52 Mindful Movement Exercises to Regulate Your Nervous System and Process Trauma is sponsored and published by North Atlantic Books, an educational nonprofit based in the unceded Ohlone land Huichin (Berkeley, CA) that collaborates with partners to develop cross-cultural perspectives; nurture holistic views of art, science, the humanities, and healing; and seed personal and global transformation by publishing work on the relationship of body, spirit, and nature.

North Atlantic Books's publications are distributed to the US trade and internationally by Penguin Random House Publisher Services. For further information, visit our website at www.northatlanticbooks.com.

MEDICAL DISCLAIMER: The following information is intended for general information purposes only. Individuals should always see their health care provider before administering any suggestions made in this book. Any application of the material set forth in the following pages is at the reader's discretion and is their sole responsibility.

ISBN 978-1-62317-981-6

1 2 3 4 5 6 7 8 9 ASIA PACIFIC 28 27 26 25 24

North Atlantic Books is committed to the protection of our environment. We print on recycled paper whenever possible and partner with printers who strive to use environmentally responsible practices.

*To anyone who has ever
experienced too much too soon*

A MESSAGE FROM THE AUTHOR:

Hello mover,

I am so glad you are here. Whether you are new to incorporating the body into healing or a seasoned professional, this card deck is here to support you—mind and body. It is a step on your journey toward healing, increasing your somatic awareness, reconnecting to your body, and liberating your mind. I commend you for your interest in movement as a catalyst for healing and your commitment to your own emotional health and well-being. I truly believe that healing the collective begins with healing ourselves—one movement at a time.

Keep moving,
Erica

DISCLAIMER

This card deck is not meant in any way to replace professional support, therapy, or medical intervention. Individual discretion is advised. If you need crisis counseling, dial 988 in the United States, or contact a crisis counselor in your area.

Contents

Introduction 1

Important Definitions and Concepts 5

Understanding Trauma 17

The Body and Trauma 23

Putting It into Practice 33

Who Is This Deck For? 37

How to Use This Deck 39

Acknowledgments 43

Notes 45

References 47

Recommended Reading 49

About the Author 51

Introduction

On July 6, 2022, just two days after the mass shooting at the July Fourth parade in Highland Park, Illinois, three miles from my home, I found myself at Highland Park High School offering crisis counseling services to survivors and anyone else impacted by the tragedy. The devastation, terror, and utter disbelief on people's faces were surpassed only by the rigidity, constriction, and tension present in their bodies. Manifesting as "deer in headlights" eyes, breathlessness in a tight chest, hypervigilance, even a frozen torso or extremity, the impact of the recent tragedy was written on everyone's bodies and represented just a few of the nonverbal signs of a nervous system in survival mode.

And it wasn't present only in the people seeking counseling, but also in the people providing the counseling, many of whom were survivors of this event themselves, trying to support their community while existing in the aftermath. Volunteers were springing into action, often unaware of how their own bodies were carrying the recent event—sometimes exhibited as busyness, witty banter, or restlessness. As the day went on, mental health volunteers began to vicariously take on postures and movement qualities displayed in the community members seeking counseling. The environment, as hopeful and supportive as it was, bred an aura of chaos and dysregulation perpetuating the state of fear and anxiety.

It became clear to me, as a dance/movement therapist, that people seeking counseling, guidance, and emotional support as well as the volunteers all had one thing in common that no one was addressing: Their nervous systems were in distress, and talking alone wasn't going to provide the support and resources they so desperately needed. Spoken language doesn't always express what we are truly feeling, especially when we can't verbalize what we experienced and how we feel. In fact, our words can deceive. We can condition ourselves to believe certain truths that are often contradictory to what our body needs and feels. We can convince ourselves, reason, and find logic with our words, but that doesn't mean it is congruent with our body's language. Immediately following a traumatic event, our minds struggle to make sense of what has happened while our brains may lack the biological ability to process and take in information. It is the body that speaks, and we must listen in order to return to a baseline of functioning and well-being. Legendary dancer and choreographer Martha Graham said, "Movement never lies."[1] When our minds struggle to grasp reality, it is the body that holds the key to being present with, moving through, and releasing our emotions.

I wished at the time of this crisis counseling that I had a body-based emotional first-aid kit, a toolbox of sorts to guide these survivors out of their heads and back into their bodies, where they could connect to the present and find some relief from the recent events replaying in their minds. I wanted to provide them the opportunity to take a dance/movement therapist with them in their back pocket, and so the idea for *The Movement Therapy Deck* was born.

Important Definitions and Concepts

To better understand the purpose of this card deck, it may be helpful to explore some key concepts and definitions.

First, **trauma-informed** means operating from a lens that is sensitive to the fact that anyone may have experienced trauma and that it isn't one size fits all. Trauma manifests differently in everyone and while there are commonalities, it is important to treat each person as an individual with their own unique lived experience. Trauma is more a question of "what happened to you?" not "what is wrong with you?" A trauma-informed approach provides a compassionate, gentle, and curious perspective on how our behaviors can be manifestations of our past experiences. It invites curiosity and exploration, while seeking to minimize the shame and guilt that often accompany trauma survivors.

Second, let's explore **somatic.** This comes from the word *soma,* meaning body. Therefore, somatic exercises are in this case movement directives with a direct focus on the body. They are experiential in nature. Experiential refers to learning that is based on experience and observation. This is a vital component of a somatic practice as it allows the body to integrate and process information through the senses. Somatic, while experiential in nature, is not experimental. These practices come with long histories passed down from generations.

Next, let's turn our attention to the word **movement.** Movement, often seen as exercise, is so much more! While all exercise is movement, not all movement is exercise. Movement is defined as a shift in posture, position, or even perspective. We have been conditioned to believe that all physical activity is good for our mental health, but that's not actually the case. Movement can perpetuate overwhelming emotions and feelings you may be experiencing, depending on how the movements are executed.

Our movement patterns are hardwired, meaning we move mostly in ways that keep us comfortable and safe. There may be a reason you are drawn to high-intensity, fast-paced workouts as opposed to meditative mindful movement. Our nervous systems get stuck in certain stress responses and our movement mirrors the dysregulation they are harboring. This is why we cannot just "calm down" or move counter to what we are feeling. We must meet our bodies and nervous systems where they are operating and then move toward security and stability. Moving in new and uncomfortable ways can cause our mind to fear for our safety, but the nervous system benefits from all kinds of movement. In fact, a more robust movement vocabulary leads to a more resilient mind and body. It is the way we engage in the new and unfamiliar movement that makes regulation possible and sustainable.

Movement affects your physical health as well as your emotional, social, cognitive, and spiritual well-being. Your movement or lack thereof influences your relationships, your personality, your interests, and your life. Furthermore, movement is not just how or where you travel in space, or even how much you exert yourself. It is how you sit, stand, gesture, sigh, breathe, exist. It is important not to just focus on why you move, but also how you move. Once you identify how you move, you can begin to understand how the way you move influences who you are, and how you feel, behave, react, and respond.

Now, that brings us to movement therapy, or **dance/movement therapy;** after all, this is *The Movement Therapy Deck*. Dance/movement therapy, as a profession in the United States, has been around since the late 1940s. It is a niche form of psychotherapy that focuses on movement, nonverbal communication, body awareness, and mindfulness coupled with talk therapy to connect mind and body and support emotional regulation by connecting with the intuitive wisdom of the body. Be advised that dance/movement therapy isn't just about dance, but rather is the core component of dance, which is movement—our body's first language.

Many people are scared and scarred by the word "dance." Dance, according to Britannica.com, is "the movement of the body in a rhythmic way, usually to music and within a given space, for the purpose of expressing an idea or emotion, releasing energy, or simply taking delight in movement itself." That is different from the art of dance, which involves performance, entertainment, and skill or talent. At some point in your lived experience, you may have been told that you "couldn't dance" based on someone else's perception or judgment of your natural rhythmic expression. This leads to suppression of not just movement, but emotions as well. Suppressing the body's natural ability and expression limits our potential and causes *dis-ease.*

Early movement experiences within the first years of life support the development of identity and self, not to mention our relationships and attachments. When we look to change or improve parts of ourselves, impacted by trauma, it is vital to revisit how these early experiences are wired in the brain and therefore patterned through the body. Trauma can intervene in or disrupt these movement patterns. Since dance/movement therapy is a psychotherapeutic approach that provides a mirror into these movement experiences, it is a discipline that supports the split of the mind from the body that occurs in trauma.

Dance/movement at its core becomes the catalyst and vessel for communication, trust, and relationship. Additionally, dance/movement becomes the means for observation, assessment, and intervention, in addition to the use of verbal processing. It is essential that the client integrates both dance and movement as we tend to the mind-body connection and bring the body into a symbiotic relationship with the mind. Dance/movement therapy supports the creation of a symbiotic relationship between the body, mind, and spirit.

As a dance/movement therapist, I don't simply tell my clients how to move. I start by inviting the possibility of movement, allowing each person to embrace the movement that is possible and already occurring for them in the moment. We move from the places inside of us that have been suppressed, buried, neglected, and ignored. The inner child, yearning for connection, validation, and love, who was made to feel inadequate, is often seen and recognized through reclaiming movement of the body. We meet the body where it is in order to guide the mind where we want it to go. Accessing what you want to feel is possible only when you know how you currently feel. Supporting where you are in the current moment through the body is necessary to healing the mind.

Therapists often refer to "meeting a client where they are," which means being present to the client's needs, not pushing an agenda, and not bringing the client into exploring or processing an experience that they are not willing, ready, or capable of exploring. While this is often the mark of a great therapist, it is not proprietary. The skill of being present to current feelings and emotions is accessible to everyone. In fact, we were all born with it. This skill often diminishes as we prioritize verbal language. *The Movement Therapy Deck* is here to provide you the support you need to get back in touch with this skill; to begin moving with intention, meeting yourself with compassion, and moving from surviving to thriving.

Think about all the ways your body changes position daily. The expansion of your lungs, the blink of an eye, every swallow—these are all ways in which your body changes position multiple times per minute. Everything your body does requires movement: digestion, immunity, reproduction—everything. The World Health Organization defines optimum wellness as "a state of complete physical, mental, and social well-being and not merely the absence of disease or infirmity."[2] To reach your optimum wellness level, it is imperative that you explore your current relationship to movement.

Movement is not just the physical shifts, but their quality. Movement can include rhythm, pace, direction, intention, tempo, shape, and size. It is these nuances and characteristics that make up our individual movement signatures, unique expressions of our emotions, thoughts, and ideas. These too are impacted in the face of trauma. Movement is not only innate to all animals, but it is our most primitive form of communication, a way to express ourselves, and a way to connect to the world around us. Our eyes are blinking, our hearts are beating, and blood is flowing through our veins. We have been moving since the moment we were conceived, as cells dividing. Once birthed, we are breathing, and our hearts are beating to their own unique rhythms. It is this breath and heartbeat that become the foundation for exploring and for connecting the mind and body. Through the mind-body connection, we can relieve our minds of the anxiety and fear that keep us in a holding pattern. Movement is not about just physical health or brain health, but also mental health. This deck is an opportunity to learn how to preserve it, protect it, maintain it, manage it, and most importantly, take responsibility for it.

It is not just the movement we *do,* but often, it is recognizing the *lack* of movement that holds the key to restoring a sense of safety, security, and stability. Movement can either be a bandaid, a quick fix or cover-up, or a soothing balm. When we mindfully and intentionally focus on movement, it becomes the medicine we all need to soothe our emotional wounds. Movement as a band-aid provides only temporary relief. This is why physical activity and exercises alone, including gentle practices, might not provide the release needed. Even yoga can trigger anxiety. Once again, it is not just the movement, but it is the execution. When we move more, we feel more, and since we carry our emotions in the body, when we move more, we have the potential to open up portals to emotions we have suppressed. Movement that acts as a band-aid is anything that supports our status quo, leading to more distraction, disconnection, and stress. When movement is used as a balm, it leads to emotional regulation, increased empathy, and self-compassion, not to mention a shift in perspective. Shifting the focus to the quality of the movement is a game changer. We begin to feel the movement from the inside out, bringing awareness to our **interoceptive** (sense of the internal state of the body) as well as **proprioceptive** (sense of where the body is positioned) senses. This deck serves as a guide to using movement as a balm, channeling you toward a greater window of tolerance as you release, dispel, and discharge trapped emotions in the body.

Understanding Trauma

You do not need to understand everything about trauma or even the nervous system to begin healing your own. I do, however, believe that it can be helpful to have some education around the neurobiology of trauma.

Housed in the body, the **nervous system** is made up of the brain, the spinal cord, and a network of nerves.

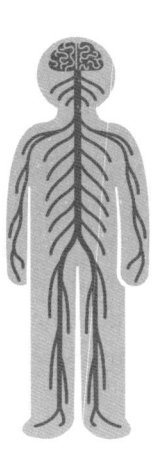

The nervous system is responsible for sending signals between the brain and the rest of the body. It supports regulation, communication, and control of the body. The nervous system contains two parts, the **central nervous system** (CNS) and the **peripheral nervous system** (PNS). The CNS is responsible for voluntary and involuntary movement, thoughts, and emotions, whereas the PNS is responsible for sensations and sensing. Within the PNS is the **autonomic nervous system,** which comprises the sympathetic and parasympathetic nervous systems. The **sympathetic nervous system** is connected to the "fight" or "flight" state, whereas the **parasympathetic nervous system** is connected to the "rest" and "digest" state. When the sympathetic nervous system is signaled or activated, heart rate increases, digestion slows or stops, and adrenaline courses through the body. When the parasympathetic nervous system is activated, heart rate slows and digestion is restored; the body is calm. The sympathetic nervous system activates when a traumatic event occurs. The activities featured in this deck act as tools for parasympathetic nervous system activation and balance.

Britt Frank, author of *The Science of Stuck,* views the sympathetic and parasympathetic nervous systems like the accelerator and brakes in a car. The sympathetic nervous system is the accelerator, while the parasympathetic nervous system is the brakes. A regulated nervous system operates smoothly between the two, whereas an overwhelmed nervous system can get stuck in a holding pattern. Somatic therapist and educator Dr. Christine Caldwell says, "Suffering originates when we try to grasp and hold still or accelerate into fight-or-flight patterns rather than experience movement that dances with what is occurring."[3] We can learn to activate the parasympathetic nervous system to reduce anxiety and stress, elevate mood, strengthen the immune system, and reduce blood pressure. This, and so much more, is accomplished through the body becoming aware of movement and sensations.

Dr. Peter Levine, creator of Somatic Experiencing, defines trauma as anything that is "too much, too fast, or too soon."[4] Frank calls this "brain indigestion."[5] Trauma, as defined by renowned addiction specialist, author, and trauma expert Gabor Maté, "is an inner injury, a lasting rupture or split within the self due to difficult or hurtful events." "Trauma," he says, "is not what happens to you, but what happens inside of you."[6] It is a response by a threatened nervous system. Maté identifies two types of trauma: **big-T trauma** and **small-t trauma**. The former is automatic responses from the mind and body in the presence of overwhelming events; and the latter is responses to culturally universal experiences such as bullying, ridicule, or inadequate connections in relationships, to name a few. They both entail "the essence of trauma," which is a "fracturing of the self and of one's relationship to the world."[7] Trauma is said to separate us from our bodies and our emotions. It distorts our reality, reframes our sense of identity and self, and limits our ability to respond to life's challenges. Since movement is an extension of the self, any change in movement impacts who we are. This is an important statement that supports just how valuable movement is when it comes to restoring aspects of ourselves that have been fractured due to traumatic experiences. Restoring movement that facilitates balance and flow, as opposed to movement that reinforces survival, is an important step in resolving and healing from our trauma.

Dr. Dan Siegel, founder of the Mindsight Institute, explains that "the simplest way of defining trauma is that it's an experience we have that overwhelms our capacity to cope."[8] This definition, while somewhat oversimplified, focuses the attention on one's inability to function or manage. This is important because when looking at how to restore functioning and widen our tolerance to overwhelming stress, movement and connection to our bodies in general are the fastest route toward enhancing our "capacity to cope."

In his *New York Times* best-selling book, *My Grandmother's Hands,* Resmaa Menakem suggests that "trauma can also be the body's response to anything unfamiliar or anything it doesn't understand, even if it isn't cognitively dangerous."[9] Bottom line is that it is an internal process that occurs to keep you alive. It doesn't mean you are broken, wrong, or damaged. On the contrary, it means your body is working, doing its job to keep you safe from threats. The problem occurs when the threats of the past continue to influence the present and future. Reestablishing safety in the body is necessary for moving through trauma. Healing must come from the body and mind to move through the events of the past.

The Body and Trauma

Trauma impacts the mind and the body in different ways. Mental or cognitive symptoms of trauma may include racing or intrusive thoughts, dissociation, negative self-talk, overwhelming guilt or shame, irritability, restlessness, difficulty concentrating, and hypervigilance. Body symptoms can include digestive or gut issues, inflammation, muscle tension, a tight chest, heart palpitations, chronic pain, and disease. But keep in mind that all mental symptoms will have an embodied component, and all body symptoms will impact your mind. This is the inherent connection between the two that is ever present even if one is unaware.

It is important to remember that everything your mind and body do in the wake of a traumatic event is meant as a means of survival. These symptoms are signs or an alarm of sorts indicating the presence of a threat, even after that physical threat has diminished or been extinguished altogether. It is your system's way of preserving and protecting itself. As Frank says, "Your brain's primary function is to keep you alive, not to make you happy."[10] Therefore, your body makes adaptations in order to survive, not necessarily to please you. Trauma poses a threat to self-regulation and as Dr. Bessel van der Kolk, author of *The Body Keeps the Score,* says, "Self-regulation depends on having a friendly relationship with your body."[11] Trauma creates a split from the self and since our identity is rooted in a connection to the body, it is imperative that we reestablish contact with the body to rebuild and reconnect to the self.

Dr. Cathy Malchiodi, expressive arts therapist, educator, and author of *Trauma and Expressive Arts Therapy,* says, "Traumatized individuals, especially those who have endured chronic traumatic events, find themselves literally cut off from their bodies, or at the very least, are not conscious of how their bodies are communicating or sensing …"[12] Traumatic events literally change our brains, but more importantly, influence how we move. Without that awareness, we remain physically stuck in patterns of nervous system dysregulation like fight, flight, or freeze. Dr. Amber Elizabeth Gray, creator of Polyvagal-informed Somatic and Dance/Movement Therapy, suggests that modifications in our movement are the foundation for emotional and psychological changes. By accessing elements of weight, space, and time—which Gray calls "portals of embodiment"—individuals can restore "a sense of belonging and meaning" after life-altering events. This is one of the many reasons that non–body-centered therapies alone do not support the restorative process, because as Gray mentions, "the imprint of fear is in the body."[13] This is a vital point because not only does trauma change the body's movement, but it can also alter our reactions when emotionally triggered.

In the face of a traumatic event, the more evolved parts of the brain responsible for processing information, perception, thinking, and reasoning go offline. This is when it is vital to connect to the lower regions of the brain, deep within the brainstem, responsible for basic elements like breath and heartbeat. These lower regions of the brain are the first to develop in the womb and are therefore considered the most primitive. If reason and logic are inaccessible due to a dysregulated nervous system or feelings of high anxiety or stress, it makes sense to change the focus from the top parts of the brain to the lower parts to facilitate self-regulation. Movement directly accesses the lower structures of the brain. Our ability to manage and cope with our emotions becomes possible not through analytical thought and reasoning, but through sensing and feeling our way through the body toward the higher regions of the brain.

Self-regulation and emotion management are associated with the limbic system, which is centrally located. It can be very difficult and nearly impossible to access those parts from the top down. According to neuroscientist Dr. Antonio Damasio, knowing comes from sensing. When we literally drop into the body, we encourage feeling and sensing from the bottom up, cognitively and physically. Only then can we restore logic and reasoning, allowing us to verbalize and cognitively process traumatic events. When we feel our way through, we can eventually think our way out of discomfort and distress.

Siegel coined the phrase "window of tolerance,"[14] meaning an optimal level of nervous system functioning that prevents us from accelerating or stopping too quickly. It is a balance between the gas and the brakes, as mentioned previously. I believe that returning to the window is not enough to thrive. We must look to widen the window, and the fastest, most comprehensive path to expanding that window is through movement.

Bonnie Bainbridge Cohen, founder of Body-Mind Centering, says, "The body is the instrument through which the mind is expressed."[15] It seems that emotional issues cannot be resolved without addressing the body that houses them. How those issues exist, live, and take up space in your body must be acknowledged, as those are literally rooted in your being. When we physically engage the body, we have the opportunity to access and rewire early developmental movement patterns often ruptured by a traumatic event. By identifying qualities of movement, you can go from "going through the motions" to embodying and expressing your emotions. We must address how the body is wired, or in some cases "mis-wired," to fundamentally rewire the mind. When we challenge our ingrained movement patterns as underdeveloped or alternative as they may be, we can navigate and rewire the psychological patterns in our minds. We can free ourselves from the fear, anxiety, doubt, guilt—everything—that keeps us from living in the moment and moving beyond the traumatic event.

All too often we minimize, deny, or numb our own experiences. When we are stuck emotionally, we always have the option to move physically. "Stuck" is just another way of saying immobile. Focusing on movement teaches the body to mobilize. However, when you are feeling frozen, stuck, or immobile, due to a traumatic event, movement can seem inaccessible and impossible.

When our body is the source of the pain and discomfort that reminds us that something horrific and unimaginable happened, or didn't happen, it can feel impossible to engage with it. Clinical psychologist and author of *The Wisdom of Your Body* Dr. Hillary McBride says that "if we cannot listen to these messages [of the body], we cannot begin to live lives of peace (because we are at war with ourselves), presence (because we are not in the here and now), and pleasure (because we are disconnected from our own sensations)."[16]

In today's world of instant gratification, it's important to remember that healing, especially through the body, cannot be rushed. Although incorporating the body into healing often accelerates the healing process, sometimes healing takes time and intention. Sometimes we need to take two steps back, dissociate, or escape temporarily to move through the pain. This is also part of acknowledging and witnessing our capacity for healing. We do not heal faster by feeling everything as quickly as possible. In fact, that can have a detrimental effect and contribute to retraumatization.

Since trauma changes not only our brains, but our movements as well, it is invaluable to work with the body to dispel and discharge the energy so we can return to an optimal level of functioning. It may seem novel, but using the body to manage and heal trauma is not a new concept. In fact, our bodies intuitively know how to support survival and safety. In our modern society of convenience, we have outsourced a lot of the movement, which means we are conditioning our bodies to override a lot of these intuitive practices designed to regulate our nervous systems amid challenging, and sometimes traumatic, situations.

The only way through it is to go into it. To release the fear, it is necessary to meet the body in its fear response. General mental health practitioners, counselors, and therapists don't necessarily receive this information in school, but are often left to educate themselves, spending countless hours and dollars reinventing the wheel. And while the field of somatic therapy is gaining traction, somatic interventions are not new. Indigenous cultures have modeled for centuries the importance of tapping into the body's inherent wisdom supporting its ability to express stagnant energy from stressful events.

This unfortunately is not an isolated incident. People all over the world are living in the aftermath of trauma—intergenerational, circumstantial, environmental, or political trauma. Regardless of how you may be personally affected by or exposed to traumatic events, or even everyday stress, the most important piece often missing from the puzzle is acknowledging the body and movement. It's important to know that the physical manifestations as previously mentioned do not dissipate simply because time moves on. In fact, without the ability to regulate our nervous systems, emotional energy can get trapped in the body, leading us to feel like we are frozen in time, unable to be present or even look toward the future. Time alone may not heal all wounds, but time spent connecting to and releasing emotions held deep within the body can.

We need resources to help us move through traumatic events that hijack our nervous systems, leaving logic and reasoning capabilities offline. When our bodies are overwhelmed and our safety is threatened, physically or emotionally, getting back to the body is a surefire way to ground, center, and stabilize a triggered mind. Recovery from trauma, specifically, is not possible until there is a familiarity with and awareness of bodily sensations.

Putting It into Practice

As with anything in life, we must practice new behaviors if we want them to become habits. Practice makes habit. This requires actively challenging and interrupting our current ingrained movement patterns. All of these somatic practices can be used in states of distress; however, it is most beneficial to your nervous system to engage in these when your system is not in crisis so that when you need to access the power of movement to calm the mind, you have these practices at your disposal. We must practice using them when we don't need them so that they are accessible when we do need them. The more we practice them, the more they become second nature. We can rely on the safety and support that come from having a steady, reliable movement practice. That safety in the body translates to emotional security and stability as well.

When we can connect to our bodies, we support the ability to connect to our emotions. Just as everyone has a body temperature, we also have an emotional temperature, a psychological homeostasis that can be achieved through becoming more aware of our body and its internal landscape. We can learn to regulate our emotional temperature through awareness practices such as those involving breath, a body scan, and mindfulness. Essentially, the more intense an emotion feels, the higher your emotional temperature. Just like our body temperature, our emotional temperature naturally fluctuates throughout the day and depends on the presence of stressors. With any stress, we can become dysregulated and overwhelmed or dissociated and checked out. Managing your emotional temperature is about regulation of body and mind. Maintaining one's emotional temperature lends itself to emotional efficiency. Emotional efficiency refers to the expenditure of emotional energy. When we are emotionally efficient, we conserve and preserve our mental health. Think for a moment of a time when you felt as if your emotions were controlling you.

When we regulate our emotional temperature, we become more emotionally efficient people, freeing up our energy for the people, places, and activities that we want to focus on. Another way I like to think of it is using a gas tank metaphor (or battery, for those of us who drive electric cars). Emotional efficiency means getting more emotional miles per gallon. We can build up reserves that allow us to manage stressors before they arise.

Additionally, when we expand our movement repertoire—all the movement at our disposal—we increase our emotional resilience. I like to call this diversification of movement. When you diversify your movement, you broaden your body's ability to access a range of emotions, as well as your ability to manage them. Emilie Conrad, founder of the Continuum Movement, said, "The more capable a system [body] is the more it's able to manage whatever comes its way."[17] You may be familiar with the phrase "roll with the punches." This is what we are training the body to do in order to create a more resilient mind. We want the body to be able to access a sense of safety in as many ways as possible.

Dr. Arielle Schwartz, clinical psychologist and author of *The Post-Traumatic Growth Guidebook,* has been quoted as saying, "Resilience ultimately allows us to embrace the unknown."[18] There is so much uncertainty in the world that we need all the help we can get to manage the inability to control everything. We can cope with the unknown by exposing our bodies to new, unusual, and uncomfortable movements—ultimately creating exposure to raw, underdeveloped, and underutilized emotions. Access to a wide range of emotions sets the stage for greater resilience, but we must find opportunities to practice feeling more and moving differently. A healthy range of motion translates to a healthy range of emotion. In the end, if we want to feel differently, we must *move* differently.

Who Is This Deck For?

While this deck can be useful for anyone who picks it up and is inspired to enhance their emotional well-being with simple somatic practices, it is intended for those feeling disconnected from the present moment and individuals seeking strategies for nervous system regulation, respite from overwhelming stress, and tools for reconnecting to the body amid dissociation. It is accessible to all ages and differing movement abilities. While not all cards are going to meet everyone's needs, there is a card for everyone. This deck is a wonderful support tool for anyone looking to reset their nervous system and increase their somatic awareness.

Trauma Survivors

First and foremost, this deck is for anyone who identifies as having survived trauma. It is a crisis intervention tool that allows the survivor to discharge the emotional energy stored in their nervous system directly following a traumatic event, situation, or trigger related to a past trauma.

Clinicians/Mental Health Practitioners/Coaches

This deck is also for those working with individuals who are seeking support around their trauma. This can be therapists, coaches, or other mental health practitioners who need body-centered exercises designed to bring clients inside their self and out of their intrusive spiraling thoughts.

Educators/Instructors

Educators need support too. This deck is a welcome addition to any classroom. Teachers can direct any student to a self-guided sensory experience when they are feeling overwhelmed, dysregulated, or anxious.

How to Use This Deck

This card deck provides a first-aid mental health kit for soothing the nervous system. Whether it is immediately following a traumatic event, supporting one's own mental health, or supporting our schoolchildren in expressing their fears and anxieties, this deck is designed to be an affordable and accessible option for anyone looking to discharge emotional stress and regulate their nervous system so they can eventually process and move through periods of intense stress, overwhelm, or trauma. I like to say that the body holds answers to questions the mind doesn't even know to ask. Especially following a traumatic event, our mind searches for answers that only the body can provide. Anytime you are unsure of what you are feeling is a time to go into the body and process or validate your own experience.

This deck is organized into four color-coded categories: Dance/Movement, Sensory, Floor Work, and Breath Work.

None of them are more important than the others, and there is no correct order in which to use the cards. While breath might seem like the place to start, it is important to meet your body where it is, regarding the energy and rhythm of your nervous system. This might mean starting with a more movement-intense card and then modulating into a still or meditative practice. Ideas of how to engage with this deck are:

- Choose one card at random.
- Create a movement practice or flow using multiple cards.
- Identify the category you are most drawn to.
- Integrate one practice into every week for an entire year.
- Use with a partner for co-regulation.

Again, there is no "right" way to use this deck, but rather the "right" way for you to support your needs and nervous system. Give yourself permission to get creative with how you use this deck. This deck is a resource, a lifeline, and a way back to the body when the mind is struggling to grasp reality.

Acknowledgments

I want to thank the wonderful team at North Atlantic Books for making this project a reality. Thank you to Shayna Keyles, Margeaux Weston, and the entire design team who made this deck come to life.

Deep gratitude goes out to my agent, Linda Konner, who continues to support my ideas and passion for shifting the way people connect to their bodies and define movement for mental health.

Thank you to my family for supporting my creative spirit and my continued growth as a mom, wife, daughter, and woman navigating the complexities and challenges of today's world.

Notes

1. Graham, 1991, p. 4.
2. Williams, 2018.
3. Caldwell, 1996, p. 16.
4. Frank, 2022, p. 56.
5. Frank, 2022, p. 57.
6. Maté, 2022, p. 20.
7. Maté, 2022, p. 23.
8. NICABM, 2019.
9. Menakem, 2021, p. 14.
10. Frank, 2022, p. 52.
11. van der Kolk, 2015, p. 99.
12. Malchiodi, 2020, p. 27.
13. Gray, 2019, pp. 147–160.
14. Siegel, 1999, p. 253.
15. Bainbridge Cohen, 2021, p. 102.
16. McBride, 2021, p. 32.
17. Conrad, 2013.
18. Schwartz, 2020.

References

Bainbridge Cohen, Bonnie. *Sensing, Feeling, and Action: The Experiential Anatomy of Body-Mind Centering.* Northampton, MA: Contact Editions, 2021.

Caldwell, Christine. *Getting Our Bodies Back: Recovery, Healing, and Transformation through Body-Centered Psychotherapy.* Boston: Shambhala, 1996.

Conrad, Emilie. "CONTINUUM: An Introduction with Emilie Conrad." Continuum Movement. 2013. YouTube video. www.youtube.com/watch?v=IAacwbfveys.

Damasio, Antonio R. *Feeling and Knowing: Making Minds Conscious.* London: Robinson, 2021.

Frank, Britt. *The Science of Stuck: Breaking through Inertia to Find Your Path Forward.* London: Headline, 2022.

Graham, Martha. *Blood Memory: An Autobiography.* New York: Doubleday, 1991.

Gray, Amber. "Body as Voice: Restorative Dance/Movement Psychotherapy with Survivors of Relational Trauma." in *The Routledge International Handbook of Embodied Perspectives in Psychotherapy: Approaches from Dance Movement and Body Psychotherapies,* edited by Helen Payne, Sabine Koch, and Jennifer Tantia, with Thomas Fuchs, 147–160. London: Routledge, 2019.

Hornthal, Erica. *Body Aware: Rediscover Your Mind-Body Connection, Stop Feeling Stuck, and Improve Your Mental*

Malchiodi, Cathy A. *Trauma and Expressive Arts Therapy: Brain, Body, and Imagination in the Healing Process.* New York: Guilford Press, 2020.

Maté, Gabor. *The Myth of Normal: Trauma, Illness, and Healing in a Toxic Culture.* New York: Avery, 2022.

McBride, Hillary L. *The Wisdom of Your Body: Finding Healing, Wholeness, and Connection through Embodied Living.* Grand Rapids, MI: Brazos Press, 2021.

Menakem, Resmaa. *My Grandmother's Hands: Racialized Trauma and the Pathway to Mending Our Hearts and Bodies.* London: Penguin Books, 2021.

NICABM. "Why Trauma Affects Some People More Than Others, with Dan Siegel." August 2, 2019. YouTube video. www.youtube.com/watch?v=yb4dgkk0kEk.

Schwartz, Arielle. *The Post-Traumatic Growth Guidebook.* Eau Claire, WI: PESI Publishing & Media, 2020.

Siegel, Daniel J. *The Developing Mind: Toward a Neurobiology of Interpersonal Experience.* New York: Guilford Press, 1999.

van der Kolk, Bessel. *The Body Keeps the Score: Brain, Mind, and Body in the Healing of Trauma.* New York: Penguin Books, 2015.

Williams, John Andrew. "The Definition of Optimum Wellness." Coach Training EDU. May 3, 2018. www.coachtrainingedu.com/blog/the-definition-of-optimum-wellness.

Recommended Reading

Marich, Jamie. *Dissociation Made Simple: A Stigma-Free Guide to Embracing Your Dissociative Mind and Navigating Daily Life.* Berkeley, CA: North Atlantic Books, 2023.

Paul, Annie Murphy. *The Extended Mind: The Power of Thinking Outside the Brain.* Boston: Mariner Books, 2021.

Selvam, Raja. *The Practice of Embodying Emotions: A Guide for Improving Cognitive, Emotional, and Behavioral Outcomes.* Berkeley, CA: North Atlantic Books, 2022.

About the Author

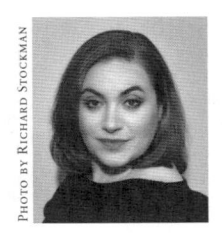

Photo by Richard Stockman

Erica Hornthal, a licensed clinical professional counselor and board-certified dance/movement therapist, is currently the CEO of Chicago Dance Therapy—the premier dance/movement therapy practice in the Midwest.

In her ten-plus years as a dance/movement therapist, Erica has worked with thousands of patients ages three through 107! Known as "The Therapist Who Moves You," Erica has truly changed the way people see movement with regard to mental health. She has been recognized by Maria Shriver's Women's Alzheimer's Movement as a woman making a difference in the fight against Alzheimer's. Erica won the 2018 Global Excellence Award in the

Alternative Medicine & Holistic Health category from Global Health & Pharma and the 2020 Social Care Award for Best Movement Therapy Center in Chicagoland from Global Health & Pharma.

Erica's area of expertise has caught the attention of multiple publications such as the *New York Times, Epoch Times, Dance Magazine, Martha Stewart Weddings,* and *Parade.* As an expert on the intersection of movement and mental health, she has appeared in hundreds of publications, podcasts, live newscasts, and radio shows, including WGN, NBC, the *Chicago Sun-Times,* the *Chicago Tribune, BuzzFeed, Bustle, Authority Magazine, Thrive Global, Medium, NBC News Better, Reader's Digest, Prevention,* and *Shape.*

Erica is passionate about working with cognitive and movement disorders, neurological conditions, anxiety and depression, and trauma. She is dedicated to bringing awareness of the field of dance/movement therapy to mainstream culture. She is eager to provide knowledge on why and how the body should be addressed in the therapeutic relationship, making the information digestible and accessible to anyone seeking to improve mental health.

About North Atlantic Books

North Atlantic Books (NAB) is an independent, nonprofit publisher committed to a bold exploration of the relationships between mind, body, spirit, and nature. Founded in 1974, NAB aims to nurture a holistic view of the arts, sciences, humanities, and healing. To make a donation or to learn more about our books, authors, events, and newsletter, please visit www.northatlanticbooks.com.